This book is dedicated to my family and friends

who struggle with weight issues.

Copyright © 2018 by the author of this book.

The book author retains sole copyright to his or her

contributions to this book.

This book, or parts thereof, may not be reproduced in

any form without permission.

ISBN 978-0-9920271-4-8

INTRODUCTION

Do you want to lose weight? Then you need to stop dieting! Seriously, you mean I can lose weight if I stop dieting? Yes, that is exactly what I'm saying! When you focus on losing weight you are facing your problem from a negative perspective. You look at food and decide what you can't eat which makes you feel like you are being deprived of something. A better way to approach dieting is to focus on eating healthy foods and living a more active lifestyle. This is a positive perspective and I can confidently say from personal experience and a lot of research, that this is a much better way to become healthier.

Weight issues were never a problem for me growing up. As a teenager, I could eat anything I wanted and never gained any weight. I was stuck at a mere 95 pounds, which wasn't unhealthy because I am only 5 feet tall. Then I had 2 children and didn't pay any attention to what I was eating or doing. I was pretty active but I continued to eat all sorts of sweets and junk food. By the time I reached age 40, I was up to 160 pounds!! This may not seem a lot for many of you, but for me, it was an additional 65 pounds that I had to carry around. My asthma got worse and I had trouble walking up stairs. I realized that I needed to lose weight so I tried a few diets that didn't work very well and I bought an exercise bike and a treadmill. I tried to stick to an exercise plan but soon I gave up because it didn't seem to be working any better than the dieting.

Then I found a booklet that was titled 'the diabetic diet'. This is a diet that consists of healthy foods that are rich in nutrients and low in fat and calories. The main focus of the diet is fruit, vegetables and whole grains. Meals are eaten in moderate amounts at regular times during the day along with healthy between-meal snacks. Meals are never missed in order that your metabolism will keep working regularly and your blood sugar will be under control. This diet can work for anyone because it helps maintain a healthy weight. You can find information about this diet on the internet and in several books or just ask your doctor.

However, before you start on any diet, you need to determine why you are trying to lose weight. If you are struggling through life with insecurities and the inability to make good choices, you won't be able to stick to a diet or exercise plan. You will just grab onto whatever comes along with a promise of success and you will end up failing and giving up. The fact is, 90% of the millions of people who diet are NOT successful. Why does this happen? It is because dieting by itself doesn't address the problem that causes us to be overweight or underweight. If you can't figure out why you have difficulty losing weight, you might need some professional help. Talk to your doctor, a dietician or a counsellor and if you have serious health or weight problems, make sure you don't start a diet without asking your doctor first. Some diets are very dangerous and could have serious consequences.

Once you discover why you want to diet, you need to create a healthy eating plan, one that includes food you enjoy along with healthy options. You also need to start exercising on a daily basis. Eating healthy without exercising is like filling your car with gas and leaving it sit in the driveway. After a while, some of the parts in your car will seize up and you won't be able to go anywhere before you have it repaired. Your body needs a good balance of proper food and exercise to be healthy and fit. Research has shown that many illnesses are linked to the food we eat and the fact that we don't get enough exercise or proper sleep. People suffer from all sorts of health issues just because they live an unhealthy lifestyle. The way we take care of our bodies has a direct impact on our health. If we don't take care of ourselves when we are young, we will probably suffer from a variety of health problems as we get older.

When you start living a healthier lifestyle, it doesn't mean that you will never be sick and it certainly doesn't mean that you won't die. But you can live a better quality of life and enjoy your days on this earth. Don't keep living with pain and misery. Stop making excuses and start making some positive changes today. Your life and the lives of your loved ones depend on the health choices you make.

In this book, I am going to try and share with you a few simple steps to losing weight and staying healthy. I hope that these ideas will help you in your search to create a healthier lifestyle and encourage you to make positive changes in your life. Since I am not a healthcare professional, I have not gone into great detail on diets and exercise plans. You should work with your doctor or healthcare professional on creating an individual diet and exercise plan that is geared directly to your specific needs.

So please stop doing those crazy diets and start losing weight in a safe and healthy way. Build your confidence, eat healthy foods and exercise regularly. I pray that God will bless you with good health!

Brenda Silveira

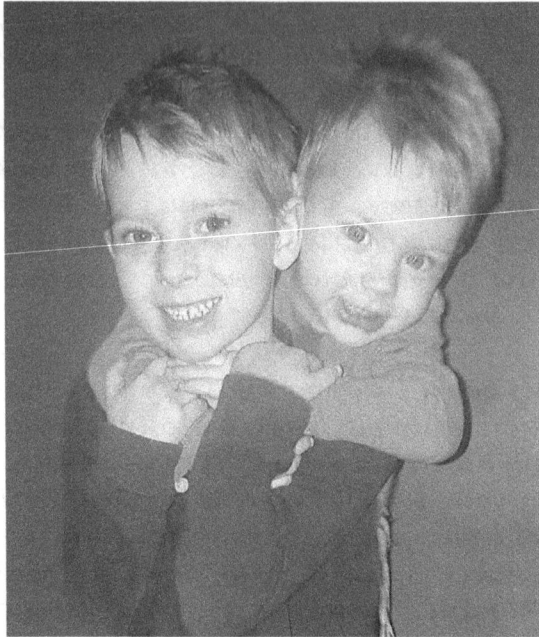

CHAPTER ONE

BUILD CONFIDENCE

The first thing you need to do before starting a diet is build your confidence. Without confidence, you won't be able to stick to a diet or exercise plan. People who lack confidence struggle through life and are unable to make good choices. This is why I tried any diet that came along with a promise of success but only ended up failing and giving up.

Confident people face difficulty with a positive perspective. They make choices that will lead to positive results. They take time to research these choices and have control over the situations in their lives. Without control, our lives end up in chaos.

Building confidence is hard in today's world. Almost everything we see and hear in the media tells us that we aren't good enough. We compare ourselves to others and feel that we don't measure up. In the search for something that will make us a better person, we fail to see our own unique abilities and strengths.

If you want to become more confident, you need to work hard on making positive changes and stop listening to what other people say about you because it probably isn't true at all. Here are some ways to make positive changes. You need to:

➢ STOP looking for the negatives in everything and start looking for the positives.
➢ STOP believing the false myths that the media is conveying to the world. Their goal is to make you feel bad about yourself so they can make money when you buy their products and services. Think about it! The media doesn't even know who we are but they are telling us how to feel about ourselves!
➢ STOP saying negative things about yourself and start using positive self-talk. Catch those negative

thoughts before they become negative words and actions.

➤ STOP focusing on what you can't do and start focusing on what you can do.

➤ STOP comparing yourself to others. There will always be someone who is smarter, faster, richer and better looking than you. It doesn't matter! Just try to be the best person you can be.

➤ STOP being around negative people and places because they will just bring you down. Instead try to surround yourself with positive people who encourage and support you and go to places where you feel comfortable.

➤ STOP worrying about all the little unimportant things in life and focus on what is important. We waste so much time on things that have no value and then we have regrets later in life.

➤ STOP getting upset when you make mistakes because everyone makes mistakes. Successful people learn from their mistakes and try harder the next time. Mistakes are learning experiences.

➤ STOP setting unrealistic goals. It is good to stretch ourselves and reach for something worthwhile but many times we are reaching for the impossible and then we think there is something wrong with us.

➤ STOP overworking and not taking the time to eat properly, exercise and get sufficient sleep. Money and power are worthless if you burn yourself out and ruin your health.

➢ STOP focusing on your problems and start focusing on solutions.

One of the things we can do to become more confident is to take control of our daily schedule and make sure that we are managing our time effectively. Nothing is more stressful than trying to do too much in a day and not having any time left to relax. Pressures to accomplish as much as possible during the day will just make us feel bad about ourselves and damage our confidence. I used to beat myself up all the time because I wasn't able to finish my daily to-do list. In reality, my list couldn't have been accomplished by 6 people in a week! That was how hard I was on myself and people do this every day, especially women. And what is the consequence? Stress related health issues and relationship problems.

Make a daily schedule or a to-do list and then review it. Prioritize it. The important things should be numbered from 1 to 5. Cross off anything that is unimportant or unnecessary. If you are rushing to take the dog for a daily walk and you have a big back yard, let the dog outside for a while and take a walk every second or third day instead. If you do daily exercise on a treadmill and also walk your dog, combine the walk and the exercise and save some time.

If there is something important that you need to do, like caring for a family member, and it takes a lot of your time, then ask for help or try to look at the situation from a different perspective. If you do something with a negative attitude, you will certainly defeat yourself before you even start. Once your schedule is manageable, you will begin to feel less stressed and you will be able to accomplish what is important. Then you will feel more confident about your life.

We can't control all the situations in our lives such as work and family obligations, but we can limit what we do. We can cut out anything that is not producing any positive results or things that are unnecessary. We need to keep our homes clean but not so clean that we can eat off the floor. If the people around you feel uncomfortable or they are afraid to make any mess, then it is time to stop being a clean freak and let some things go. Leaving a bed unmade or a few dirty dishes in the sink is not a major issue if you are stressing yourself out trying to keep things perfect. Your health is more important than a perfect home. Besides, there is no such thing as perfect in an imperfect world. So stop pushing yourself to do the impossible!

Laughter is an excellent way to help boost your confidence and bring peace into your life. Research has shown time and time again that laughter reduces stress and brings healing to the body. Try to find situations where you can engage in laughter and laugh whenever you can. Being able to laugh at yourself when you do something wrong is a good way of releasing your emotions.

Of course, there are times when you need to cry about a difficult situation and that is okay. Crying is a normal reaction and it is healthy to allow yourself to release stress in this way as long as it doesn't happen continually. God gave us emotions as warning signals and we should never suppress or ignore them. Instead we need to embrace them and learn how to use them in a healthy way.

Anger is a good example of an emotion that warns us something is wrong. Anger is actually a secondary emotion. Typically, fear or sadness is underneath the anger and we have to discover what is causing us to be angry. We should never hold anger inside and not deal with it but we should also not take out our anger on other people. It is important that we learn how to deal effectively with any negative emotions so they don't cause any lasting damage to ourselves and others.

Simplify your life. If you are doing too much, it will take away your joy. You don't have to be a super-person and do everything. If you are too busy, you won't have peace in your life. Don't fill your life with possessions and activities. Spend time doing the things that are important. Cut back, cut out. Get rid of anything you can live without and spend less time with people who drag you down.

Always try to control your thoughts as they will influence how you live. If your thoughts are negative, they will stop you from enjoying life. Be consciously aware of what you are thinking and change any negative thoughts into positive thoughts. A good way to do this is to keep a journal and write down your daily thoughts. Then you can look at them and change any negative words to positive words. If you actively work on changing your thoughts you will soon develop a habit of positive thinking.

Weight issues are often the result of psychological issues and this can result in poor habits and eating disorders. We may have been hurt in some way and we use food to feel that we have control of our lives. Before starting any kind of diet we should first determine why we have unhealthy eating habits.

Consider these questions:
- Did you grow up in a family that had healthy or unhealthy habits?
- Were you encouraged to eat or forced to eat?
- Did the adults in your life set a good example or a poor example?
- Was there peace during mealtime or a lot of stress?

- Why do you eat junk foods?
- Do you eat when you are unhappy or alone?
- Do you continually snack between meals?
- Do you feel satisfied after eating or are you hungry right after you eat?
- Does eating help you cope with life better?

All of these are signs of a deeper problem that is using food as a substitute for other needs. Food can be used as an escape and a denial that you have a problem. Or it can be a control issue if you are lacking control in other areas of your life. If you are really struggling, you should talk to someone you trust so they can put you in touch with someone who can help. This could be a family member, a friend, your doctor, a pastor or a counsellor. Don't deal with a serious situation alone. As long as you continue to deal with your problems alone, you will never be free from any guilt or pain.

Never feel that you are stuck and nobody can help you. Nobody in this world is ever beyond help and there are always kind and caring organizations and people that offer assistance. Prayer can help tremendously. God can reach right down into the deepest pit and lift you up. He can work through the people around you to get you back on a healthy path.

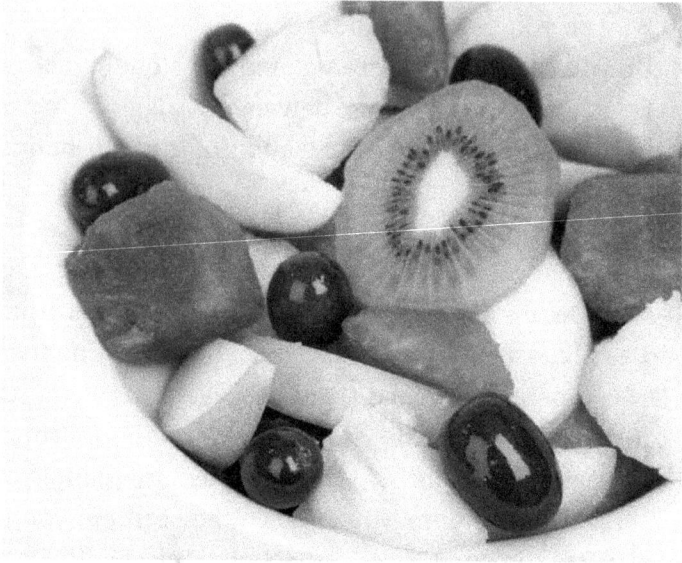

CHAPTER TWO

EAT HEALTHY

A proper diet is absolutely necessary for a healthy body. The statement, 'You are what you eat' is so true. Sadly, many people today have terrible eating habits because they feel insecure about their body image and believe they can only be happy and successful if they maintain a certain body weight.

Did you know that there are over 100 million people just in the United States who are on a diet and that these people spend over 20 billion dollars on diet books, diet drugs and weight loss surgeries? You are just one of millions of people in the world who are trying to lose weight.

Every day we are bombarded with conflicting messages from the media. We see ads that promote irresistible, unhealthy foods and scrumptious, high calorie desserts which we buy and eat, resulting in weight gain. Then we see ads that promote weight loss products and services, which make us feel guilty about eating too much so we try all sorts of diets and ways to lose weight. When we fail, we turn to food again to soothe our pain and the cycle continues. We have to get into a routine of focusing on healthy eating instead of focusing on constant dieting.

However, before you attempt any diet or exercise plan, you should talk to your doctor or health care professional, especially if you have any major health concerns. You need to make sure you are eating foods that will benefit you and doing exercises that will not cause any further problems to your health.

When dieting we need to lose weight slowly and steadily. Our body doesn't like drastic changes so it will store fat and become resistant to weight loss. A realistic goal is to lose 1-2 pounds each month. Some diet plans will make you believe that you can lose a lot of weight in just a few days or weeks. Seriously? We didn't gain weight in a few days or weeks so how can we fall for that ridiculous lie? If you want a diet to work, it takes time and patience. Quick weight loss can be very dangerous to our bodies.

What we put into our bodies can either make us healthy or unhealthy. In order to work properly, our bodies need food that is nourishing and sufficient. We need to eat 3 proper, relaxing meals every day. Skipping meals or eating on the run is not healthy.

Anyone can develop healthy habits. When we were born we didn't crave pizza and pop. We learned these unhealthy eating habits from our environment. Children who are often given candy as a reward for doing something right, can become addicted to sugar. Children who are offered fruit and fresh vegetables as a snack and only have candy as a special treat, are more likely to develop healthy eating habits.

God gave us pure foods that were intended to make us strong and help us live a long, healthy life. Man has tampered with God's perfect foods, adding chemicals and stripping them of vitamins and minerals. With all the processing, many foods have become dangerous to our health.

There are so many choices as to what foods we can eat today, however many of them are unhealthy and full of toxic poisons that can actually destroy our health. Toxic wastes and poisons build up in our bodies when we eat too many processed foods. The body will naturally try to eliminate the toxins but it can't get rid of all of them. This causes our bodies to become weak and sick. Then disease comes. We can get chronic infections, stomach problems, aches and pains or just feel plain lousy all the time.

If we want to feel good, we have to eat proper foods. The only way to healthy dieting is having a proper, balanced diet. This requires a complete change in the way we think about dieting. We need to re-train our brain to focus on healthy eating instead of focusing on weight loss because it is a negative approach to dieting. This can be accomplished by building new habits and working hard to maintain them every day. Just focus on healthy eating today and don't think about tomorrow, next week or next year. Setting long-term goals is important but if you focus on the future, it will be hard to get through today. Set short-term goals that you can reach every day and then you will achieve your long-term goals. If you set your mind to eating healthy first thing every day, it will become a well-established habit in a few weeks. Healthy eating keeps you feeling full and you won't be craving junk food. Do it today, then do it tomorrow again and the next day again. You can get through 'one day' and pretty soon, your 'one day' will be an accumulation of weeks and months.

Healthy foods include fruits, vegetables, grains, nuts and seeds. People who are struggling with poor health can often regain their health by changing their eating habits. By putting the proper nutrients in our bodies, it helps repair any damage that has been done through eating improper foods. Many of us eat unhealthy for years before we notice any serious problems. Our blood can become clogged and our body starts breaking down causing serious health issues like heart problems, stroke and diabetes. If we don't take notice and start changing our lifestyle, we will continue to feel worse and could have an early death.

When you eat healthy foods, you feel better and you will have a much better attitude about life. Food can do a lot to improve your attitude and control stress, anxiety and depression.

There are many diets available today and it can be confusing to people who are trying to lose weight and stick to a diet plan. Many of these diets are not healthy and are very restrictive. Sometimes you can lose weight but you might also be losing something else that you need to be healthy. You can lose energy, important nutrients and even your confidence when you are unable to reach your goal.

Instead of constantly dieting and trying to find something that works, we should be focusing on eating healthy foods. The fact is, there is a huge failure rate for people who diet. As I mentioned in my introduction, 90% of people who diet do NOT lose weight and often gain back more weight. The media does such a good job of making us believe that we can look better, have more friends and be more successful if we use their diet or exercise plan. Ads on TV and in magazines are purposely created to make us feel bad about ourselves so companies can make a lot of money through our pain.

Young people are especially pressured because they are trying so hard to measure up to others and be accepted. If they lack confidence in themselves, they believe that dieting will help them become popular and successful. Also, many parents unknowingly pass down insecurities about their own self-image in their personal struggle to maintain a healthy weight. When a parent or other role model is always dieting and obsessing about their looks, it is pretty much a guarantee that their children will follow their lead, especially young girls.

Parents need to teach their children the importance of eating healthy foods and how it will benefit their physical, mental, emotional and spiritual health. If parents are strong in what they believe and set a good example, their children will often accept the same view and live a healthier lifestyle.

If you are trying to set a good example and keep your family eating healthy, don't bring certain foods into the house. The person who buys the groceries is helping create habits for everyone. Junk foods will likely get eaten and bad habits will be formed. Make sure you keep a good supply of healthy snacks in your fridge and pantry. Put things out in containers on the cupboard so they can be easily seen and readily accessible. When people want to snack, they will grab what is easily available so make sure there is always something healthy at eye level.

When you start a new diet, don't try to change everything all at once. Introduce 1 or 2 new healthy foods every week and eliminate 1 or 2 as much as you feel comfortable. Trying to change everything all at once can frustrate you and cause you to fail.

If you feel like you are not reaching your goals and you have been eating unhealthy foods, don't beat yourself up and **don't give up**. We all fall off the horse sometimes but we just have to get back in the saddle again and take control of our lives. If we want to feel good, be strong and have energy, we need to eat simple, healthy foods. Before you start eating, say a simple prayer of thanks. Then eat slowly and try to relax so your food will digest properly.

Eating healthy does not have to negatively affect your social life. If you are invited to someone's home for a meal and you know that they serve unhealthy options, offer to bring a salad or veggie tray and then just go and enjoy. Eat small portions and be polite but don't feel that you have to eat everything they offer. You can also go out to eat and enjoy a meal. Many restaurants today have healthy options. Even fast food restaurants have salads but try to avoid these places as much as possible. If you crave french fries, enjoy them once in a while as long as you don't do it on a regular basis.

Family get-togethers can be difficult when you are trying to eat healthy. Often there are lots of yummy foods to enjoy that are high in sugar, salt and fat. Just keep your portions small and don't overeat. If there are 3 desserts, you don't have to eat them all. Select a small portion of the one that appeals to you the most and savour it slowly.

If you don't eat proper foods every day, you should consider taking vitamins. Just make sure they are natural and don't have any added chemicals. Check with your doctor as to what would benefit you. However, don't rely on vitamins to provide you with all the nutrients you need. They don't take the place of eating proper foods.

In the next chapter I am going to discuss some ways that you can create healthy eating habits. If you start implementing some of these ideas, you will be well on your way to becoming a healthier you!

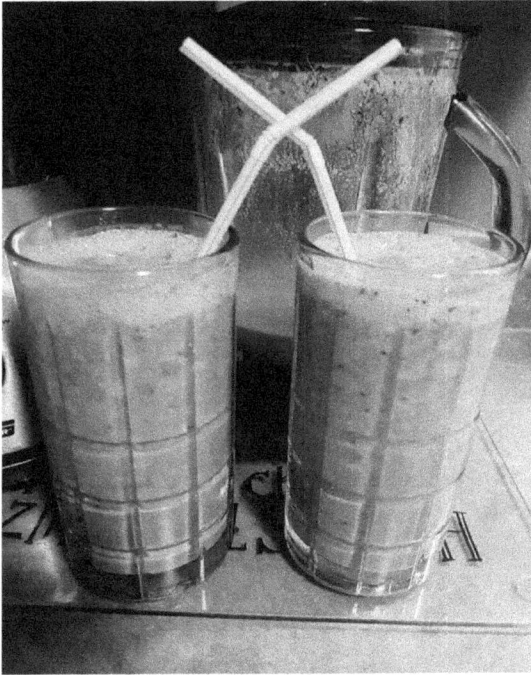

CHAPTER THREE

HEALTHY EATING HABITS

Dieting can make you feel bad. Healthy eating makes you feel good. You will lose any excess pounds and maintain a healthy weight. The only successful way to diet is to change our eating habits. All habits are learned so if you put your mind to it, you can develop healthy eating habits. Nobody is born with a desire for cheesecake and chocolate cookies. We can acquire a taste for almost anything, so it is important that you develop healthy eating habits so you can be a good example to your children by teaching them how to eat healthy while they are still young.

Did you know that food can heal you? Sometimes it can even reverse health problems or at least slow them down. Food is fuel for your body just like gas is fuel for your car. It would be really foolish to fill your car with garbage because it wouldn't run properly. So why do we fill our bodies with garbage? We are much more valuable than a vehicle!

Here are some ideas that can change your eating habits.

Create a list of healthy foods and plan meals in advance. Make a grocery list and don't pick up things that are not on the list. **Never** shop for groceries when you are hungry or in a rush as you will pick up all sorts of things you don't need and probably shouldn't be eating. Poor choices are made when you are under pressure. Always make sure that you check what is in the foods you are eating. If the label contains all sorts of information you don't understand, then you probably shouldn't be eating it.

Be more positive. If we have a negative mindset, we will make poor choices. We will give in to unhealthy cravings and give up on ourselves too easily. Developing a positive and realistic perspective is the key to developing a healthier lifestyle. You ARE worth it and you CAN be successful!

Don't skip meals. When we skip a meal, our bodies think we are heading for famine and it will fight back by storing fat. Breakfast is the most important meal of the day and one we should never miss. During the night our metabolism slows down while we sleep. Food provides the necessary fuel to speed it up so it can burn calories during the day. Having a full stomach will give you energy and also help you make better choices. If you don't want to eat a full breakfast, at least eat some fruit or make a smoothie.

Eat smaller portions and have a healthy snack between meals. When we eat large meals, the glucose levels in our bodies rise which leads to low blood sugar. Having 3 proper meals a day in smaller portions will keep our bodies in balance and burn calories more evenly.

Eat slowly and chew food well. It takes about 20 minutes for our brains to tell our body that it is full. If we rush through a meal, our food will not be digested properly and our body will feel hungry and stressed.

Never overeat. It is so easy to overeat at a buffet. All that scrumptious food just waiting to be tasted! I would

25

literally eat until I was sick and then I felt lousy for hours. When we overeat, our digestive system has to work harder than it should and it puts excess stress on our bodies.

Eat lots of fresh fruit and vegetables. Research has proven that a diet rich in fruit and vegetables has a huge impact on your health. Eat a variety of types and colours to provide your body with the mix of nutrients it needs. Eat them raw, steam or bake and don't overcook them as it takes away all the important minerals and vitamins. Always keep plenty on hand and put them where you can see them.

Garlic is an excellent choice as it has antifungal, anti-inflammatory and antibacterial properties. It can also help lower cholesterol and regulate blood pressure and blood sugar levels. Chop and use in your favourite recipes for meat, pasta and dips.

Eat whole grains. White flour, white rice and white bread are popular but not healthy. Buy whole wheat flour, brown rice and whole grain bread. If you have trouble getting used to the different taste, try mixing them together in slowly increasing measure. Instead of 1 cup of whole wheat flour, use ¾ white and ¼ whole wheat. Do the same with the rice until you get used to it, then keep increasing until you are no longer using white.

Choose poultry, lean meats and fish. Chicken and turkey breast are healthy choices. Eat fish 2–3 times a week as this will help lower your cholesterol. Salmon (fresh or canned), tuna (fresh or canned), sole or lake trout are excellent choices.

Choose low fat dairy products. Skim milk and low–fat yogurt are best. Buy eggs direct from a market or local farmer as they are fresher. Cheese is high in salt so eat in moderation especially if your blood pressure is high.

Choose organics. Many of our foods are treated with dangerous pesticides. Organic foods are usually safer as they are free from harmful chemicals, have more nutrients and they taste better. They can be a bit more expensive but isn't your health worth it? Besides if everyone bought organics, it might force other companies to change the way they grow their products.

Eat foods with fiber. When we eat foods with high fiber, it lowers our cholesterol and reduces the chance of heart disease and diabetes. It also aids in digestion and helps us feel full so we don't overeat. We should consume 25 to 38 grams of fiber each day to maintain proper functioning of the digestive system. However, the average adult eats only 15 grams of fiber or less! Beans are a rich source of soluble and insoluble fiber.

Eat unsalted nuts and seeds. These are great for snacking between meals and will help cut any cravings you may be experiencing. Almonds are an excellent choice but only eat a handful because nuts are high in calories.

Avoid sugar and sugar substitutes. Too much sugar can cause diabetes, tooth decay, hypoglycemia and even lead to mental problems and learning disabilities. Sugar substitutes are also dangerous because of the chemicals in them.

However, we do need to treat ourselves once in a while, so have a small piece of pie or cake, a little chocolate, one scoop of ice cream or other yummy sweet! A good time to do this is when you have reached a goal. Just make sure you don't celebrate with too many sweets or you will gain that weight right back again. Raw honey is a good alternative to sugar. It has also been found helpful in reducing allergies, relaxing a cough and soothing a sore throat.

Avoid fried foods and fast food. They taste good but are high in calories, fat and often salt. They raise bad cholesterol, lower good cholesterol and are linked to heart disease and diabetes. Enjoy them once in a while but don't make it a regular part of your diet.

Avoid eating out as much as possible. There is nothing nicer that enjoying a good meal at your favourite restaurant. However, your meal will probably be high in fat, sugar and salt as it makes the meals taste better. Look for healthy options like salads, vegetables, fish and lean meats.

Carry healthy snacks with you in case you get hungry. If you are always rushing from one place to another, it can be very hard to eat healthy. Preparing food takes time and sometimes we just have too much to do to think about our next meal. Fast food places, corner stores and vending machines can look very appealing when you are hungry. Instead of taking a chance on filling up with unhealthy foods, pick up some food bars, low fat crackers or cookies, some fruit and unsalted nuts. These can easily be carried in a purse, backpack or even in your vehicle for those times when you feel hungry or know you will miss a meal. Never leave yourself open to temptation.

Cut back on caffeine. Caffeine is a stimulant that can cause health problems when consumed in high quantities. Coffee, tea, chocolate, soft drinks, energy drinks and even some medications contain caffeine. Although research has shown some positive benefits from caffeine, it also shows several negative benefits. Try switching to decaf or cut back to 1-2 cups a day.

Cut back on salt. Use in moderation as too much salt can result in serious health concerns. We need some salt in our bodies and it adds flavour to food, so don't cut it out completely. It is never necessary to put salt in any baked goods. I have never put salt in any recipe for pies, cakes, cookies or other desserts and they always turned out really good without any salt.

Avoid processed, canned or frozen foods. Many foods today are over-processed so they look appealing, last a long time and are easy to prepare. However, processing strips all the vitamins, minerals, enzymes and rich nutrients from foods along with the taste. Then salt, sugar, toxic fats and chemicals are added to preserve the food for a long period of time.

Most of all, be patient. Nothing worthwhile is ever gained by being impatient. Society pressures us into doing thing quickly and getting immediate gratification. This is not realistic or attainable. Take your time, be persistent and you will reach your goals.

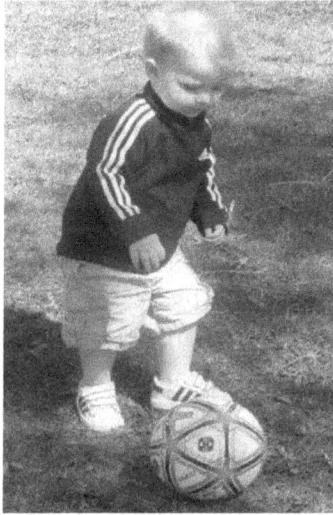

CHAPTER FOUR

EXERCISE IS IMPORTANT

Exercise is a word that we don't like and the sad fact is that many of us never exercise. We live in a world that has an increasing rate of health issues including obesity. We all know the benefits of exercise but we avoid commitment because it takes time and energy. However, if we want to be in good physical shape, we must have regular exercise. Without proper exercise our physical, mental, emotional, spiritual and relational health will suffer. Unhealthy people usually make unhealthy choices in all areas of their lives.

Picture a beautiful garden overflowing with colourful flowers and in the middle of that garden, there is a fountain with a running waterfall. So lovely to look at! Now, what if the owner decided it was too much trouble to look after the garden and turned off the water to the fountain. It wouldn't take long before those amazing flowers and bushes were dead and ugly weeds took over the garden. The water left in the fountain would soon become stagnant and dirty. Without proper and continuous care, the garden would not be so lovely to look at any longer. Just like a garden, we need to provide our bodies with proper and continuous care.

What kind of activity do you do during the day?
Do you sit more than you move?
Does laundry and cleaning wear you out?
Do you stay in bed as long as you can?
Are you out of breath going up and down the stairs?

If 'yes' is the answer to any of these questions, you are probably out of shape and need to start exercising. Our bodies were designed to move so we can stay in good shape, however, today many people move as little as possible.

For centuries people were constantly on the move and they were a lot healthier. Before people had cars and public transportation, they walked almost everywhere and got lots of exercise. Today people drive most places, even to the corner store! Machines have replaced a lot of jobs that required manual labour and now many people sit and work or do a minimum of walking. We often sit for hours watching TV or using the computer. Then we make things worse by eating unhealthy snacks. Instead of walking down the street to chat with a neighbour, we can just text them or use social media. These are certainly not ways to benefit our bodies or our minds. We need to get on our feet and exercise. Just make sure you check with your doctor first if you are dealing with health issues.

The benefits of exercise are numerous. Here are a few:
✓ Lessens stress
✓ Helps control blood sugar
✓ Reduces possibility of heart attacks, stroke, cancer and other illnesses
✓ Alleviates pain
✓ Reduces depression and anxiety
✓ Slows down aging
✓ Promotes weight loss
✓ Increases energy
✓ Builds strong bones
✓ Improves digestion
✓ Helps you sleep better
✓ Can help reduce chronic pain

One of the best and cheapest exercises is walking. Always wear comfortable clothing and shoes and walk in a safe location. Swimming is also a good activity. I find that exercising in a pool is easier than exercising on land and it gives you a double benefit because of the water pressure.

Other fun ways to keep fit are cycling, dancing, hiking and playing sports. Make sure you start slow and build up activity so you don't get worn out and give up. 5–10 minutes per day to start is good especially if you have health issues. Once you feel comfortable with that time, increase your activity up to 30 minutes at least 3–5 times per week. Don't plan to exercise right after a meal or right before bedtime as it will interfere with digestion and keep you awake.

Find someone to exercise with you. Having a partner will encourage and energize you. This can also help build strong relationships. Make sure you rest if you get too tired. Pushing yourself too much can be harmful to your health. Skip a day if you don't feel well and rest so you are ready to go again the next day.

Lifting weights is also very beneficial for your body. This will strengthen your muscles, increase your metabolism and burn fat. Start with 2 pound weights and increase if you are able. Don't lift anything heavier than you can comfortably manage. If anything starts to hurt, then stop.

I keep a basket beside my sofa with items that I can use to exercise while watching TV. It has weights, theraputty, a theraband and a heating pad in case I need it. If I experience pain, I stop and take some deep breaths, then use the heating pad.

If you work in an office or somewhere that requires a lot of sitting, you can even fit some simple exercises in to your work day. Stand up and stretch. Lean down and touch your toes. Stretch out your arms and make circular motions. Do pushups on a wall. Take the long way to the bathroom. After lunch take a short walk. Use the stairs instead of the elevator. Be creative! You might even encourage some of your co-workers to move with you.

Even if you are older or in poor health, exercise can benefit you. I am a senior and I exercise more than I did when I was younger. After 2 strokes, I have learned how important it is to keep moving. Exercise has brought back strength to my arms and legs and helped relieve my back pain and chronic sciatica. If you are confined to a wheelchair, there is wheelchair yoga and other exercise programs that can help. Find out what is available and get moving!

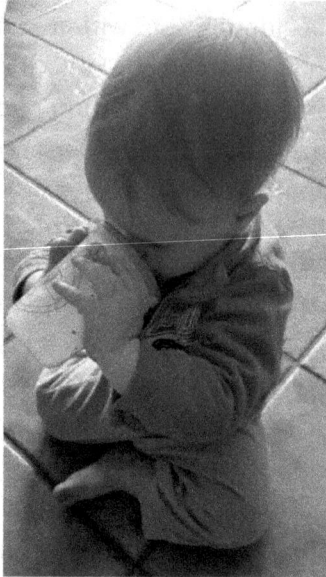

CHAPTER FIVE

THE IMPORTANCE OF WATER

Water is the most important nutrient our bodies need. We can go a few weeks without food but we can't last more than 5-6 days without water. Every day our bodies lose about 2 quarts of water which needs to be replaced or we will become dehydrated.

When we feel thirsty, our body is telling us that it needs water. If we lived our entire lives and only drank water, we would be a lot healthier and we would certainly save a lot of money that we spend every day on a variety of drinks. Besides that, when we get sick, medical care can be very costly. It is actually much cheaper to stay healthy.

Unfortunately, many people don't like the taste of water, so they rarely drink any, filling up instead on juice, milk, soft drinks, coffee, tea or alcohol. None of these will provide us with the benefits that water does. Instead we will end up with a variety of ailments such as: headaches, digestion problems, joint aches, constipation and skin problems.

There are many benefits of drinking water:
✓ Lubricates joints and helps prevent arthritis
✓ Makes skin smooth
✓ Reduces effects of aging
✓ Makes immune system more efficient
✓ Prevents clogging of arteries
✓ Helps prevent memory loss
✓ Improves digestion
✓ Aids in weight loss

Another way to help keep your body hydrated is eating lots of vegetables and fruits. They contain water and have various other health benefits also.

How much water should you drink? Try to drink at least 6 eight oz glasses per day. If you drink a glass of water about 30 minutes before a meal, it will cut your appetite and help you lose weight. Drink a glass between meals and one before bedtime unless you have reflux or another health condition that would interfere with your sleep.

Don't wait until you are thirsty to drink water because at that point your body is already feeling dehydrated. Make a habit of drinking water several times a day.

Encourage your children to drink water. Children don't always realize that they are thirsty and can become dehydrated quickly especially if they are playing sports or during hot weather. Get them into a healthy habit at a young age and help them avoid serious health issues in their future.

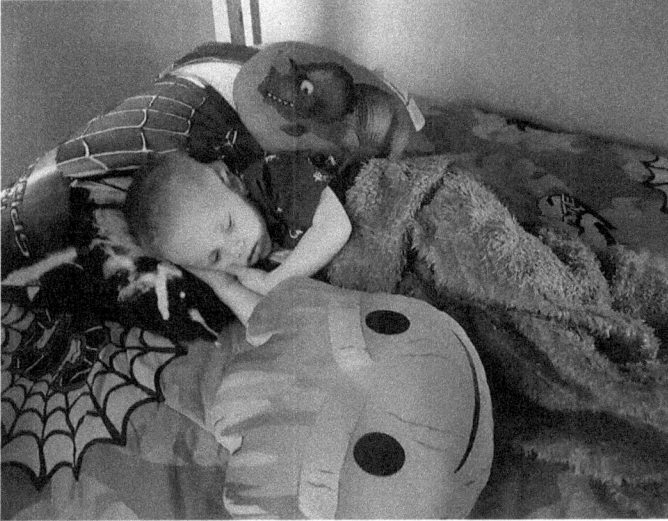

CHAPTER SIX

REST & RELAXATION

Sleep is very important for good health. During the night, or whenever you sleep, your body is being repaired, restored and recharged. Your mind takes a break from all the stresses of the day and gets ready to start again the next day. When you don't sleep well, it affects your health in a negative way. Millions of people suffer from sleep disorders and feel tired most of the time. Many take sleeping pills in the hopes they will sleep better.

People who don't get enough sleep can have health problems and safety issues including:

- Chronic fatigue
- Depression and anxiety
- Inability to concentrate, easily distracted
- Making poor choices
- Poor work habits and less hours worked
- Higher risk of accident or injury
- Poor reaction time when driving or operating machines
- Weight gain
- Heart disease and stroke
- Diabetes

Adults should get at least 7 to 9 hours of sleep each night in order to have good overall health. If you have difficulty sleeping, here are some ideas you could try:

- ➤ Don't drink caffeinated drinks in the evening
- ➤ Avoid cigarettes and alcohol
- ➤ Don't eat heavy or sugary foods in the evening. A light snack is okay unless you have digestive problems.
- ➤ Don't exercise too close to bedtime
- ➤ Don't watch anything that is violent or scary. Listen to some quiet music or read a book.
- ➤ Make sure you have a comfortable mattress and pillow
- ➤ Keep your bedroom dark and quiet
- ➤ Use a fan or white noise machine

- Don't turn on lights if you get up to use the bathroom. Better to use a night light instead.
- Don't keep watching the clock. If it is lighted, have it turned away from you.

You also need time during the day to relax and unwind especially if you are always on the go. Working people are often busy with home and family obligations and they leave little time for themselves. Everyone should take at least 30 minutes per day to just relax and do something they enjoy like reading, meditating, writing or just doing nothing.

A daily nap can be helpful for anyone who lives a stressful lifestyle. Just a 30 minute nap can help you feel better and full of energy so you can get going again.

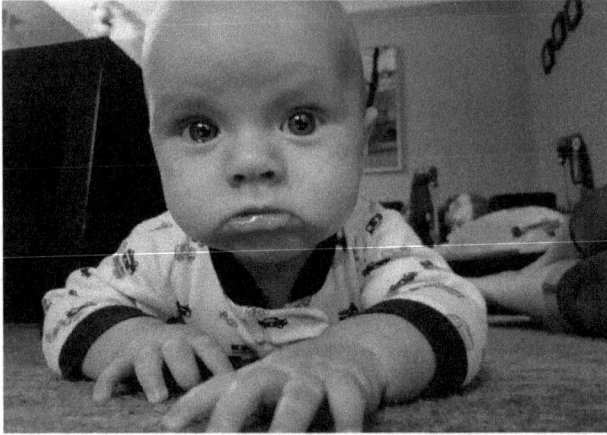

CHAPTER SEVEN

HOW STRESS AFFECTS YOUR HEALTH

Stress is a huge barrier to losing weight. If we have a lot of stress in our lives, we will never be able to eat healthy and exercise effectively. People that are over-stressed often turn to food for comfort. They grab fast or frozen foods when they are in a hurry and eat so quickly that their food doesn't have time to digest. When time is short, they often miss meals because they don't allow time to eat.

Stress is a normal part of life and it affects our lives in either a positive or negative way. Positive stressors can energize you and move you forward in life. Family events like a wedding or a new baby can bring you joy and peace. Other positive stressors can warn you of danger, like having a vicious animal coming your way or the feeling you are being followed. This warning gives you a chance to avoid the danger or to make any necessary changes.

Negative stressors on the other hand can literally suck the life right out of us and cause physical and emotional problems. These can include depression, anxiety, weight gain or loss, high blood pressure, heart attack, stroke, faster aging and even death. Sleep is disrupted leaving us exhausted and irritable and we find it very hard to relax. We are easily angered and find it hard to control our emotions.

Negative stressors can include things like:
- High and/or unrealistic expectations
- Conflict in relationships and marriages
- Financial issues
- Job problems
- Family pressures
- Continuous driving in heavy traffic
- Living in a noisy, busy location
- A cluttered home
- Unforgiveness and holding onto grudges
- Misunderstandings
- Speeding through life with no breaks
- Illnesses, injuries

Some people don't even realize that they have too much stress in their lives. If they have grown up in families that push themselves to overachieve and expect the same from their children, they will think this is the way everyone is supposed to live. They become adults who believe the lie that the busier we are, the more value we have.

How many times do people ask us how we are and we reply, 'Busy'. We expect so much of ourselves that it is impossible to live up to our own expectations. Multi-tasking has become '*a badge of honour*' and of course we all want to feel important. But sadly, all this activity is not benefiting our bodies. Instead it is taking a toll by robbing us of good health.

Therefore, since it is impossible to eliminate all stress from our lives, we need to learn how to control it.
Following is an idea that I came up with to help you deal with stress. I call it the '**STRESS**" method.
Stop what you are doing.
Take note of the situation in a journal or notebook and outline the cause of the stress.
Review your notes. Do this later in the day when you can sit down quietly by yourself. If you are too emotional, you won't see the situation clearly.
Evaluate your reaction. Was it proper, logical, realistic? Or did you blow the situation way out of proportion? Write down your answer.

Situation – can it be changed, minimized or eliminated? Yes? No? How? Write down your answer.
Set up a plan of action for the next time this situation come up. Write it down so you can refer to it and deal with it in an effective way.

Every time you feel stressed, try to take the time to stop and write down the situation. Just stopping yourself for a few minutes to think before you react, can even lessen the stress and help you make better choices. If you don't have access to your journal, use your phone or tablet and copy it to your journal later. Then take a few minutes at the end of the day to review your notes and make a plan of action. You will soon see a pattern emerging as to what situations cause most of the stress in your life.

Another thing that is important and that can also help reduce stress is natural light. We all need to be outside in the sun and the fresh air. Sunlight is like medicine and can heal your body. It manufactures Vitamin D, helps heal wounds by killing germs, helps depression and calms nerves. We should try to get outside as much as possible all year round as it will benefit our health. Always dress appropriately for the weather and when it is very hot, make sure you avoid being in direct sun for too long.

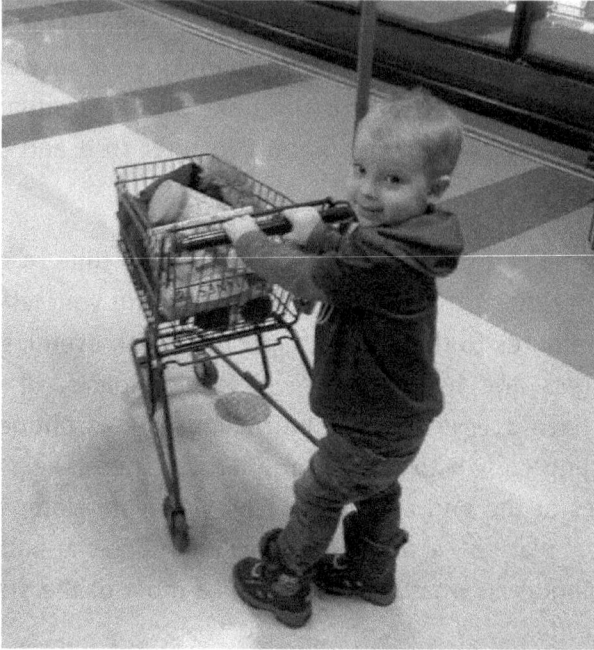

CHAPTER EIGHT

YOU CAN BE A HEALTHIER YOU

There is no magic formula that will immediately help you lose weight and become healthy. If you want to be healthy, you have to work hard and be patient. Some people can lose weight more easily than others because we are all different, but it will still take time.

Be careful what you put into your body because everything has consequences. You may not feel bad right away but unhealthy eating can damage your body on a long-term basis. What you eat and how you treat your body will determine how healthy you will be in the future. You have the power to become fit and stay healthy. All it takes is eating healthy foods, exercising daily and minimizing your stress.

Create a daily journal and keep track of your progress. Write down what foods you will eat the next day and choose a time that you can exercise. When you do the action of writing things down, you are more likely to follow through. When you have completed your daily goals for food and exercise, check them off. Draw a happy face if you have been successful! However, if you don't reach your daily goal, don't feel discouraged. Try again the next day and don't give up on yourself.

Your body is valuable and nobody can take care of it except you. Treat it with respect and make good choices every day. Pray for guidance and surround yourself with people who love and support you.

You CAN be a healthier you! Develop a positive perspective and look after yourself!

PERSONAL NOTES

PERSONAL NOTES

ABOUT THE AUTHOR

Brenda Silveira, the Author of The Caterpillar to Butterfly Self-esteem Workbook is known for inspiring people while building their confidence through her workshops, blogging and Confidence Coaching.

Her first book in the series called "**Grandma's Notes**" is named **Grandma's Notes on Parenting.** It gives empowerment to new parents by highlighting a few simple ways to raise children in a positive environment. Brenda's candid recollection of her own lifetime of struggles helps individuals to realize they are not alone.

Her second book in the series named **Grandma's Notes on Dieting** provides a realistic approach to healthy eating.

Brenda, a graduate of Stratford Teacher's College, a Girl Guide leader, Guide Commissioner and former owner of a housekeeping and yard maintenance company, is also the creator of I M Confident Niagara Canada, a project that promotes confidence through a website that has information and visual presentations. Be inspired by Brenda's writing by visiting www.imconfident.com.

www.ingramcontent.com/pod-product-compliance
Lightning Source LLC
Chambersburg PA
CBHW060646280326
41933CB00012B/2174